10 Da

Complete Natural Detox Guide with Herbs

The Complete Natural Herbal Guide to the 10 Day Detox

By: David A. Grande

PUBLISHERS NOTES

Disclaimer

This publication is intended to provide helpful and informative material. It is not intended to diagnose, treat, cure, or prevent any health problem or condition, nor is intended to replace the advice of a physician. No action should be taken solely on the contents of this book. Always consult your physician or qualified health-care professional on any matters regarding your health and before adopting any suggestions in this book or drawing inferences from it.

The author and publisher specifically disclaim all responsibility for any liability, loss or risk, personal or otherwise, which is incurred as a consequence, directly or indirectly, from the use or application of any contents of this book.

Any and all product names referenced within this book are the trademarks of their respective owners. None of these owners have sponsored, authorized, endorsed, or approved this book.

Always read all information provided by the manufacturers' product labels before using their products. The author and publisher are not responsible for claims made by manufacturers.

Paperback Edition

Manufactured in the United States of America

DEDICATION

This book is dedicated to all those who struggle to lose weight and keep it off. Not all options work for all people but it does take dedication and willpower to stay the course when an option is found.

TABLE OF CONTENTS

Publishers Notes 2

Dedication 3

Chapter 1- Herb And Herbal Matters - An Overview 5

Chapter 2- Cooking With Fresh Herbs 9

Chapter 3- Herbal Medicine- Regulations And Research 12

Chapter 4- "Medicinal" Herbs Can Be Harmful.............................17

Chapter 5- Chinese Herbs- Research And Advancements 21

Chapter 6- Herbal Detox And Weight Loss.................................24

Chapter 7- Herbal Tea And Weight Loss 26

Chapter 8- Herbal Detox Herb- Echinacea 29

Chapter 9- Herbal Detox Herb- Fennel Seed 31

Chapter 10- Herbal Detox Herb- Marigold Flowers 33

Chapter 11- Herbal Detox Herb- Milk Thistle.............................35

Chapter 12- Herbal Detox Herb- Spirulina.................................37

Chapter 13- Herbal Detox Herb- White Sage 39

About The Author..41

CHAPTER 1- HERB AND HERBAL MATTERS - AN OVERVIEW

For many years man's existence has been inextricably linked with the wild herbs and plants that grew naturally in his environment. Irrespective of color, creed, religion or country we have all turned to these natural resources to add to our food or use for medicine. We have even learnt how to cultivate these herbs amongst other plants to protect and stimulate their growth.

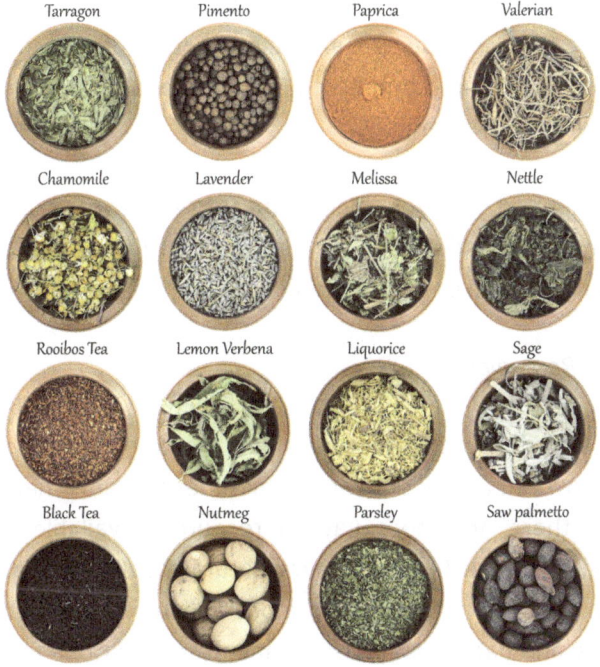

But in our headlong rush into the future we should not discard the knowledge so carefully gleaned over the centuries.

Herb and Herbal Matters will help point you toward this knowledge. Whether your ambition is to grow an herbs garden indoors or a pot of chives on your kitchen windowsill, whether it is to cultivate a container of medicinal herbs or plant a formal herb garden, my aim is to help you.

Even if you are not interested in cultivating your herbs then I'll introduce you to some of the world's most popular herbs and herbal supplements.

Herb Garden

If you have the enthusiasm and the room, you can create a small herbal garden that can be both particularly productive as well as visually stimulating. If you don't wish to cultivate a dedicated herbal area then consider the amazing results you can achieve with introducing herbs as companion plants growing alongside your other flowers and vegetables.

If space is limited then you might want to consider the practicalities of growing herbs indoors or a windowsill garden using traditional compost cultivation or a hydroponics medium.

Medicinal Remedies

In today's modern world there are new treatments and medicines being discovered all the time and sometimes it seems that we have forgotten there are more natural resources available to us as remedies. Over the last few years natural health remedies have begun to make a resurgence as more and more people look for alternative and natural ways as our ancestors had done for treating illnesses and diseases and increase their understanding of the power of medicinal plants and herbs.

These time served remedies offer an alternative that has proved to be believable and viable to large numbers of people across the globe.

For centuries natural herbs and supplements have been part of the curative and preventative medication of cultures around the world. Their reported low risk and minimal or no side effects are attractive benefits to those who believe that the commercially available drugs are too potent.

Natural herbs offer access to an ancient knowledge of vitamins, herbal supplements and natural herbal remedies to cure and prevent an unhealthy life.

Herbal Tea

It is reputed that tea, next to water, is the most frequently drunk beverage around the world. Part of this popularity is because of the antioxidant values they carry; partly because herbal teas are credited in providing the body with protection against free radicals and partly because they just taste so darn good.

Herbal tea remedies have been used, and refined; throughout history soothing and treating a wide variety of aches and pains and helping people regain the balance in their lives.

Unfortunately in the global markets of today buying herbal teas is not as straight forward as it should be. You must identify that the quality of the ingredient used is paramount – they must not be bulked up with irrelevant plant parts.

Chinese Herbs

Some call these folk remedies, others herbal treatments, whatever they are called their continued and refined use over the last tens of hundreds of years means there is a knowledge of natural healing sources which should not be dismissed.

10 Day Detox Diet

The Chinese have a simple and time honored use of herbal remedies. Simplistically theirs is a holistic approach, believing that cures as well as prevention comes about through diet, exercise and the balanced ingestion of herbs. The Chinese theory holds that herbal and dietary treatments can restore and maintain the body's balance.

CHAPTER 2- COOKING WITH FRESH HERBS

The beauty of living with, and cooking with fresh herbs is that they offer multiple benefits. We are all aware of the breadth of their legendary health benefits, giving relief to the illness of man, animals and plants alike. But are you aware of just how wide the choices of culinary herbs are that can also impart their health benefits whilst sparkling up our meals?

By applying a little knowledge and common sense we can combine the taste offered by numerous herbs to enhance our food and drinks; whilst making sure we get the medicinal benefits each fresh herb has to offer.

Preparing Natural Herbs For Cooking

The first thing that needs to be said is that cooking with fresh herbs offer a greater potency in taste and health benefits than dried or frozen herbs. If you can grow them yourself in your own herb garden, then that's the best of all. Herbs should be thoroughly washed and dried before use. If you are using a large quantity of natural herbs, treat them as you would salad greens, washing them under running water and drying them in a salad spinner.

Use about twice as much fresh herb to dried herb to get the same balance. But preparation could not be easier. Finely chopped or minced your herbs (unless the recipe dictates otherwise) and add to the meal shortly before it finishes cooking. Overcooking natural herbs can lessen the flavor and remove valuable nutrients.

Medicinal Properties Of Common Natural Herbs

Now we turn to the health benefits of some of the natural herbs most commonly used in cooking.

1. **Dill** is rich in dietary fiber and calcium. It is also a digestive aid and appetite stimulant. The emperor Charlemagne used to provide it at his banquet table for the benefit of guests who had eaten too much.

2. **Sage** is a renowned herb with many beneficial uses and is valued highly as a cooking herb and as a medicine to help keep you healthy. Sage is used as a medicinal treatment for over perspiration and has a strong anti-bacterial property; it is used in some mouthwashes to inhibit gingivitis and other problems of the mouth.

3. **Rosemary** contains vital antioxidants that can help to eliminate free radicals in the body, lowering the risk of cancer. It may also help relieve nasal congestion.

4. **Oregano** is a natural antiseptic and painkiller. The oil found in its leaves was historically used to treat pain and infections, being almost as powerful as morphine.

5. **Evening Primrose** is an astringent, antispasmodic, anti-coagulant, reduces high blood pressure, stimulates liver regeneration, and anti-arthritic.

6. **Basil**, that other great standby of Mediterranean cookery, has antacid and anti-gas properties. It is also a mild sedative, so be wary of using fresh basil in breakfast and lunch dishes. At supper time, on the other hand, these sedative properties can be an advantage, as they will help you sleep when it's time to go to bed.

Almost any aspect of cooking can be improved with the careful addition of herbs. Nearly all aspects of cooking can be enhanced by introducing herbs into the preparation process and cooking with fresh herbs present more problems in doing this than using dried herbs. You simply need to cut up the herb or herbs add seasoning,

David A. Grande

if required, and add to your meal 15 or 20 minutes before you serve. It's important that you don't add the herbs too early in the cooking cycle as they will lose their potency.

CHAPTER 3- HERBAL MEDICINE-REGULATIONS AND RESEARCH

The use of herbal medicines in the USA is less widespread than in a majority of developed nations. The key reason for this is that their distribution has mostly been limited to health food stores, which are patronized by only a small proportion of the population. Despite the lack of market coverage, sales of herbal medicines are estimated to be growing by around 15% a year.

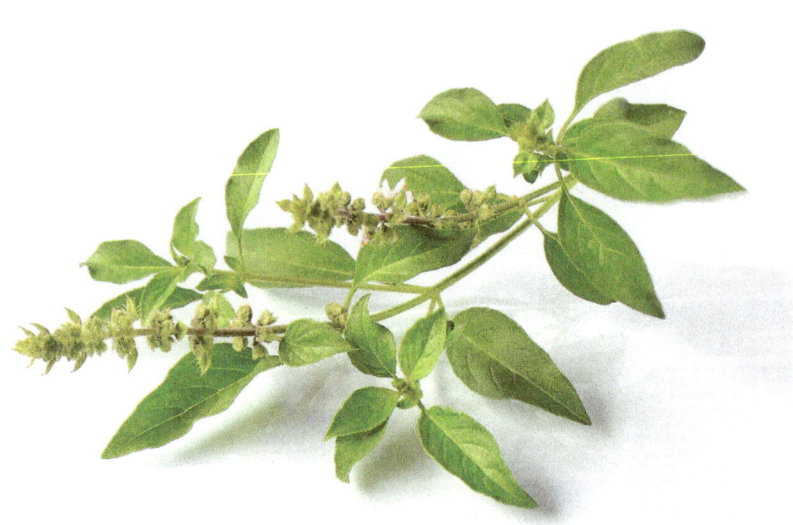

The US Food, Drug and Cosmetic Act passed in the late 1930's has been a major reason for restraining sales, in that any products that claim to treat, cure, mitigate or prevent a disease must be licensed in the same way as allopathic drugs. Most natural products in the USA are regulated as foods or food additives. As such, most regulatory action occurs in areas of safety. Under this scheme, herbal products are assigned a Generally Recognized as Safe status as long as recognized experts say they are safe and are not contradicted by other experts with opposing evidence. However, there are some exceptions to this rule. These are the better known herbs which were listed by the US Food and Drug Administration for OTC (over the counter) status. Following a review of OTC drugs by the FDA, most of these drugs were dropped because of a failure by the US herbal manufacturers to submit evidence to support their use as OTC products.

The FDA has introduced regulations specifying that dietary supplements must provide scientific evidence for any health claims that are made on the label. How this move will affect the sale of herbal products classed as dietary supplements remains to be seen.

The use of herbal products as prescription medicines is dependent on whether the relevant country's licensing legislation evaluates the product as it would a "chemically purified ingredient" or whether it treats it as a separate class of product. In countries such as Germany and China, the requirements for licensing a plant extract as a prescription drug are made simpler because historical information on its use is considered pertinent. In most other countries prescription drugs made from plants must be evaluated for safety, efficacy, and quality.

Therefore, the majority of herbal medicines are sold OTC and it is this sector that is generating the greatest growth. The level of control in this area varies considerably, and seems to have a correlation with the strength of the sector in each country. However, the major problem faced by herbal medicines is their acceptance by the medical profession.

Herbal Supplements

Some of the most commonly used herbal supplements are echinacea, garlic, ginkgo, ginseng, St John's wort and valerian. All have indications relevant to the health of the older patient.

The issues for herbal medicine and herbal supplement use by the older patient are, as for any age group, effectiveness, safety, and potential for interaction with prescribed medication. Healthcare in older patients focuses on management of chronic conditions; most require multiple drug therapy. It has been suggested that the average older adult takes five prescription drugs every day; thus particular care is needed with herbal supplements.

The most common use of Echinacea is as an herbal supplement for prevention and treatment of respiratory infections, although it is also taken as a general immune booster. However, a Cochrane review of echinacea use for the common cold was inconclusive. A large trial investigating preparations of E angustifolia for rhinovirus infections found no clinically significant effect on cold symptoms. Adverse effects with echinacea are rare but include allergic reactions and GI complaints.

In recent years, garlic has been the focus of serious medical and clinical investigation as herbal supplement regarding its role in cardiovascular-related factors. A review based on 45 trials concluded that, compared with placebo, garlic may lead to small reductions in total cholesterol, LDL and triglyceride levels at one to three months. Studies have investigated the effects of Asian ginseng (Panax ginseng) and Siberian ginseng (Eleutherococcus senticosus), the herbal supplements used on physical and psychomotor performance, cognitive function, immunomodulation, type II diabetes, cancer and herpes simplex infection, but have shown no definitive evidence of effectiveness for any of these conditions. Due to the potential adverse effects of

David A. Grande

both ginsengs (insomnia, anxiety and manic symptoms) neither can be recommended as a supplement for the older patient.

Depression may affect up to half of older people. St John's worth is mostly used to treat mild to moderate depression and evidence for its effectiveness is undisputed. The herbal supplement Valerian is used to treat both insomnia and anxiety. Trials suggest it does have hypnotic effects above those of placebo and may be as effective as oxazepam for sleep disturbance. However, the quality of the studies is mixed and it is difficult to be definitive about its effectiveness. Adverse effects reported are headache and GI upsets. Valerian should not be taken with other sedative, hypnotic, or CNS depressants.

Use of herbal supplements is a question of choice. If done properly, it can lead to a sense of empowerment and control over an individual's health care. Good communication between patient and health care provider is essential to ensure safety and maximum benefit.

If you wish to go ahead with herbal supplements, take note of the following:

1. **Research before you buy** - Whether herbal supplements are right for you will depend on the herb and your health and medical history. Like over-the-counter and prescriptions, supplements have active ingredients that can affect the function of an individual's body. Talking with a doctor and researching the product are recommended when considering taking any supplement.
2. **Practice safety**- The Food and Drug Administration oversees the safety of food and drug products in the United States, but they do not include approval of herbal supplements. Product labels usually include certain

information such as its name, quantity and contacts for the maker, packer or distributor.

3. **Pick the right supplement**- Amid the limited government regulation on herbal supplements, consumers are advised to consider only standardized supplements, buy single-herb products, and use extra caution with imported medicines.

4. **Find out if you should avoid supplements**- People who should avoid herbal supplements include anyone taking prescription or over-the-counter medications, expectant or breast-feeding mothers, anyone planning for surgery, or younger than 18 or older than 65.

5. **Talk it over with your doctor** - A physician can give details about specific herbal medicines that might be appropriate, potential side effects and interaction with current medication taken, and alternatives such as lifestyle changes, through diet or exercise.

David A. Grande

CHAPTER 4- "MEDICINAL" HERBS CAN BE HARMFUL

People have always treasured herbs and spices and have gone great lengths for them. Witness the magi, the Polo family and the British East India Company. It's not that different today. (Finding the medicinal herbs and spices that launched a thousand caravans centuries ago is not always easy in) The hardest to find are spices sold in bulk and fresh green herbs.

A word of explanation first; or rather two words: "Herbs" and "spices" are not the same thing. Although some people use them interchangeably, the definitions are different in culinary use. Herbs are seasonings made from the fresh or dried leaves of plants (such as parsley, sage, rosemary and thyme). These are mostly known as medicinal herbs. Spices, however, are made from other plant parts, such as seeds (mustard), berries (juniper), bark (cinnamon) or bulbs (garlic) and often ground or powdered. And yes, under such a rule, dillweed would be an herb but dill seed a spice.

Although many supermarkets carry a variety of bulk foods, the biggest selection remains at a handful of health food stores. Stocks range from oreganos to hard-to-get medicinal herbs such as golden seal and orris root. For these storekeepers, the spice trade is as redolent of exotic places and global interplay as it was for London merchants waiting for their ships to come in centuries ago.

Many of those who specialize in medicinal herbs prefer them in their most natural state. Medicinal herbs come from organically grown plants and have not been irradiated; when possible, it is preferable for these plants to have been growing wild. Finding freshly cut green herbs for cooking or garnish has always been more difficult; the best alternative often was to grow your own.

Page | 17

Although some supermarket chains carry fresh basil, dill, rosemary and cilantro, finding crisp parsley often is a chore.

The first medicinal herbs were produced during the Renaissance, grown in physic gardens behind monastery walls. In the Elizabethan era, the herb garden became part of the landscape pattern. Many of the herbs used in cooking today throughout the world - such as coriander, rue, sage, savory and thyme - still come from the Mediterranean region, and their names attest to their continuous cultivation for over two thousand years.

Through every stage from seed to harvest, medicinal herbs fit into any garden picture. In a rock garden or in the crevices of a wall garden, Chamomile (Matricaria chamomilla or Anthemis nobilis, babonag in Hebrew), basil (Ocimum basilicum, reihan), savory (Satureja hortensis, star) and thyme (Tkhymus vulgaris, koranit) are very suitable. These and others make a rock or wall garden much more interesting.

Generally speaking, the poorer the soil, the better the medicinal herb. The best conditions for a successful herb corner are a sandy soil (with some lime), sun, and good drainage. Ideally, an herb garden is small. It can even be part of the flower garden or, where there is sufficient space, in the vegetable section. It can be a small rectangle or triangle against a background of other plants.

If there is a pool in the garden, or a damp, more-or-less shady spot, mint (nana) should be planted. It is best to plant it separately, because its grasping roots spread rapidly. One can buy medicinal herb seed packets from seed shops or nurseries. Sow them in small containers filled with light soil. Styrofoam strawberry flats from the greengrocer are ideal. Water with a small watering can or a hand-sprayer. Most medicinal herbs originate in warm climates and are used to infrequent rainfall. Never over-water your plants, as that will rot the roots. Inspect the containers every morning, and water them when the soil feels dry.

Stroll down the aisles of a local health-food store and you'll find a cornucopia of herbal products - teas to relax your nerves, and capsules of chamomile, parsley and marshmallow. Armed with a good herbal guide, a person may be able to ease such common ailments as nervousness, gas or a sore throat with herbs in capsule or tea form.

But while the secrets of herbs for medicinal purposes have been handed down for generations in some families and cultures, the use of some herbs may be harmful; among them are germander and comfrey.

The risks of herbs got new attention recently when a study conducted in France found that six women and one man who had taken daily doses of germander, an herb touted as promoting weight loss, developed liver inflammation. This acute hepatitis receded once the germander was discontinued. Although the seven took the recommended doses of germander, the authors of the report in the Annals of Internal Medicine, cautioned that "controlling the safety of herbal medicines is particularly difficult, because they are self-prescribed."

In a check of several local health-food stores, germander, a member of the mint family, did not appear to be well-known. But in an editorial accompanying the study, the writer noted that germander is often mislabeled and sold under the name scutellaria or skullcap.

Concern about the use of herbs, minerals and vitamins has prompted the Food and Drug Administration to conduct toxicity studies of the products. Part of the problem surrounding herbs are a plethora of books that sometimes contain inaccurate information

10 Day Detox Diet

and FDA regulations that do not permit manufacturers of herbs to make claims for the products.

Below are the guidelines for reducing the risk of herbal poisoning:

1. Do not take herbs if pregnant, trying to become pregnant or if nursing.
2. Do not give herbs to infants or children.
3. Do not take a large quantity of any herbal preparation.
4. Do not take any herb on a daily basis.
5. Buy only preparations that have the plants listed on the packet (not a guarantee of safety, but better than nothing).
6. Do not take anything containing comfrey or germander.

CHAPTER 5- CHINESE HERBS-
RESEARCH AND ADVANCEMENTS

Comprehensive research and clinical applications have proved that henbane, a Chinese herb first used 2,000 years ago in china, can cure many illnesses hitherto hard to cure, according to "guangming daily".

In the past 30 years Chinese medical circles have put forward many views on the curative properties of Chinese herbs. In 1983, xiu ruijuan of the Chinese academy of medical sciences discovered that henbane was effective against thrombus and made an important breakthrough in the study of microcirculation.

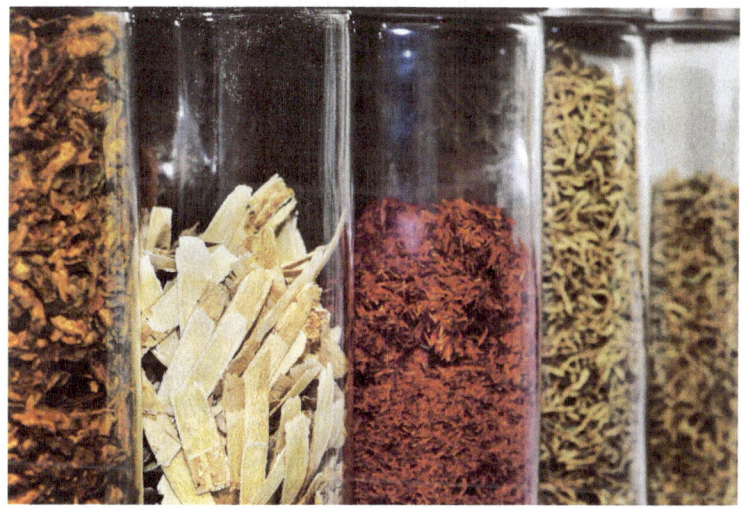

The Chinese micro-circulation and henbane research society was set up in 1979 and has over 2,000 members. Research on the Chinese herb henbane has advanced from clinical observation to basic theory. It is now being used in hospitals in large and medium cities. A henbane medicine center to combine research, clinical use and production is in the preparatory stages. There are now over ten factories producing henbane medicine.

Another Chinese herb approved by health authorities helped cure the 150 million Chinese children suffering from anemia. One of the doctors who developed the medicine called it syrup for invigorating the spleen and strengthening energy. It has proved effective among 90 percent of 5,000 children suffering from anemia, and the Beijing public health bureau has given it the thumbs up. Around 50 percent of China's children suffered from anemia caused by improper dietary habits and congenital deficiencies. Children in many developing countries suffer from the disease.

The Heilongjiang province in China has greatly improved the supply of herbal medicines by protecting resources and expanding the cultivated area. Short supplies have been reduced from over 100 varieties a few years ago to 77. Heilongjiang has now 25 conservation zones covering 2,800 hectares for rough gentian (gentiana scabra), fangfeng (saposhnikovia divaricata), Chinese thorowax (bupleurum chinense), rhizome of wind-weed (anemarrhena asphodeloides) and gorgon fruit.

There are 12,000 peasant households specializing in production of medicinal herbs on about 800 hectares. As a result, some Chinese herbs, which had been on the verge of extinction, such as slender acanthopanax (acanthopanax gracilistylus) are again thriving.

So, with the popularity of Chinese herbs, it is no surprise that the pharmaceutical giant, Upjohn signed a research agreement with the Shanghai Institute of Materia Medica for screening and development of compounds derived from ancient Chinese herbal medicines. Upjohn received research quantities of compounds isolated from 10 Chinese herbal medicines and will pay the institute a specific sum for access to the most promising of these compounds. The compounds, which have not been studied in the

David A. Grande

West, have been used for centuries in herbal preparations in China for treatment of a wide range of disorders, including cancer, cardiovascular disease and malfunctions of the central nervous system. If any commercial products are developed as a result of the agreement, Upjohn will also pay royalties to the Shanghai Institute, depending on product sales.

CHAPTER 6- HERBAL DETOX AND WEIGHT LOSS

With celebrities and ordinary people joining the trend of using herbal detox diets to get rid of unwanted fats and extra pounds, it is good to understand how this approach can help people and what benefits they can offer to the human body in general.

First and foremost, herbal detox diets use all natural ingredients so the unhealthy toxins that have accumulated in your body for many long years will be driven away. For a weight loss regime to be effective, you need to understand what your body needs to achieve and what herbs can truly help you accomplish your weight loss goal.

To have a clear picture of what herbs really work for an effective detox diet and what would suit your body's requirements, take a look at the list presented below:

1. **Apple cider vinegar** helps to increase the metabolic rate of the body. With this ability, it can lower blood cholesterol levels and reduce body fat, thereby preventing the body from storing unwanted fats.
2. **Soy protein** can provide your body with its energy requirements and you will tend to eat less because it can leave your stomach feeling full even with just a minimal food intake.
3. **Green tea** is not only good in eliminating body toxins. When you take green tea regularly, you will have an increased metabolism and at the same time, it can also suppress your appetite for food.
4. **Psyllium seeds** have been used extensively by women who want to lose weight. Because it is an effective appetite

suppressant, you will find yourself eating less, yet feeling fuller every time. And as seen in actual tests, you will see the seeds swell when placed in a glass of water. This property is the reason why you have a feeling of fullness even with a lesser food intake.

These are just some ideas that can aid a successful detox diet. So instead of spending hundreds and thousands of dollars on products just to achieve a slimmer and healthier body, you have a more affordable option that will also produce amazing results when used well. And if you want to ensure that the detox diet you are going to try is safe for you, you can always ask for a professional opinion first before jumping into anything.

CHAPTER 7- HERBAL TEA AND WEIGHT LOSS

Like the rest of us you've no doubt heard of the seemingly remarkable reputation of herbal tea remedies that cure all ills. But just how true is it?

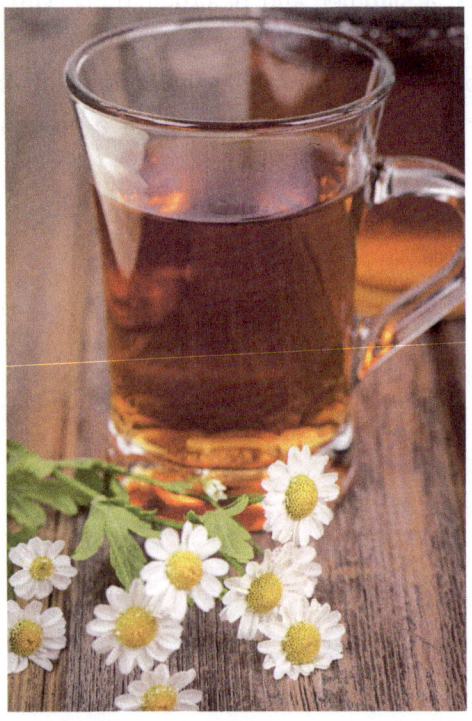

Most evidence that I've been able to find is anecdotal. That is to say it's quite subjective. However, in saying that I've also discovered that if the subject is approached in the right way. If you stop and think about what you are doing and listen to sound practical advice then there is a world awaiting you that is bursting with health benefits and flavors.

David A. Grande

Of course none of the reputed remedies should ever replace a conventional medical practitioner but you can improve your health if you include herb tea regularly in your diet. Some of the things you can cure with herb tea are a cough, a cold, constipation, depression and even obesity. That's right; you can even lose weight if you regularly drink herbal tea throughout the day.

Can't Stop Coughing? If you can't stop coughing, you'll be happy to know that there are herbal teas just for you. A cough can really ruin your day. You have that tickling in the back of your throat, and you cough to get rid of that. You soon find that you're coughing every few minutes. This makes your throat raw, you begin to get sore in your stomach and it's very miserable. A tea made for coughs will soothe your throat and get rid of the tickling in the back of your throat so that you can go about your day once more without having that irresistible urge to cough.

Now we all know there is no cure for the common cold whether you have one with or without the dreaded cough. So how can drinking herbal tea make you healthier?

Well this claim is often substantiated because it is recognized that herbal tea will help strengthen your immune system, thus helping your body fight off those bad germs and infections and help speed up recovery. Not only that, but a good tea will rehydrate you which is perfect for anyone who isn't feeling so well.

For constipation, a natural laxative tea is just what the doctor ordered. Drinking good herbal tea remedies for this purpose and you'll soon find that you no longer have to hold everything in so to speak. You'll feel better, your system will be working more regularly and you won't be feeling so full and bloated.

Puffy eyes? Inflammation? Need a new hair shampoo? Some herbs have the unique properties or being able to be used as teas, poultices and tinctures. The chamomile herb is one such champion and is recommended in all three of these examples.

Today we are all fixated with body weight – Obesity!! So can herbal teas help us in this area?

It's true that a good herb tea will help you lose weight. Drinking this tea will flush your system and that will help remove the fat. You should also eat correctly and exercise but the herbal tea will help you feel full faster, will hydrate your system and will help you feel better and thinner than ever.

Now I would like to reiterate how potent I have found herbal teas. But I do not rely on them wholly to help my physical and mental well-being! I would strongly urge you to follow suite, you should always see the doctor if you're not feeling well They are the only ones who are going to be able to give you an in-depth and authoritative diagnoses of any aliments you may feel are affecting you.

Use herbal teas wisely and they will always help you feel well again and ready to face any challenge.

CHAPTER 8- HERBAL DETOX HERB- ECHINACEA

Lately, more and more women have joined the trend of using the natural way of detoxifying the body through herbs. Let us now take a look at Echinacea for detox so you can have a better understanding of how it can cleanse the body of the accumulation of toxic substances and speed up the disposal of unwanted waste.

What Is Echinacea?

Echinacea may not be a very familiar name to many, but you may have heard the common names used to refer to this herb. It is also known as red sunflower, black Sampson, Sampson root or narrow-leaved purple coneflower.

Why Is Echinacea Good For Detox?

Echinacea is a highly recommended detoxification agent due to its cleansing and rejuvenating properties. Although it is not known to have a direct detoxifying action, it has proven its use as a tonic for overall cellular rejuvenation.

Where Can You Find Echinacea?

Echinacea, a perennial flower, is native to the eastern part of the North American region. The flowers, leaves and roots of the Echinacea plant can be used for detoxification purposes. Its effect can be maximized when mixed with myrrh, marigold and golden seal.

Products Containing Echinacea

The most common products that use Echinacea as an ingredient include:

- Zinc Echinacea syrup
- Echinacea capsules
- Echinacea herbal supplements
- Echinacea teas

The Best Ways To Use Echinacea

Aside from the popularity of Echinacea as an ingredient for solutions used in the prevention and cure of colds, it is also best used in the natural detoxification of the body. For a tea mixture that uses Echinacea for detox, it would be best to mix it with sarsaparilla root, red clover, milk thistle and dandelion.

On a precautionary note, this mixture should not be taken by someone who is pregnant or nursing. It is also not advised on people with uterine or breast cancer, autoimmune disease or gallstones.

David A. Grande

CHAPTER 9- HERBAL DETOX HERB- FENNEL SEED

Fennel, scientifically referred to as Foeniculum vulgare, is a plant that is native to the Mediterranean shores. It has also become naturalized on river banks and coastal areas in many parts of the world. It is largely used as an herbal detox agent because it is great for cleansing the liver and clearing uric acid build-up in the joints. The seeds of the plant are used for detox purposes. Other names used to refer to the plant include Florence fennel, carosella, finocchio, wild fennel, sweet fennel and large fennel.

What Does Fennel Seed Do?

Being a natural diuretic, fennel seeds act as a helpful tonic for the kidneys and help settle the stomach. It can flush out toxins from liver and kidneys resulting in improved performance of these vital organs. It tastes good when taken as tea and safe for pregnant women and children. It is available in the market in syrup, powder, tincture and capsule form.

When Do You Need Fennel Seed?

Fennel seed is highly recommended for people who want to lose weight because it can help reduce appetite. Another remarkable benefit that one can get when taking fennel seeds is the removal of toxic wastes from all body parts. It can also aid the process of digestion, remove gas, provide a calming effect to the nervous system and kill harmful pinworms.

Fennel seeds are mostly used for body detoxification and colon cleansing because it has been found that the herb can increase perspiration and urination. These are the two major ways by which toxins are purged out of the human body.

How To Use Fennel Seed?

Optimal detoxification and body cleansing can be achieved by drinking one cup of fennel infusion three times daily. It is prepared by putting one teaspoon of fennel seeds in a muslin pouch and steeping it in 6 ounces of boiling water for a period of three to five minutes. Then release a stronger flavor of the fennel seeds by squeezing the pouch gently.

More and more shops now also sell ready-made fennel tea bags.

Fennel Seeds For Slimming?

Traditionally, fennel seeds were known as a slimming herb because of its remarkable ability to stimulate metabolism. It can also help dissolve stored fats and repel water retention. During the early stages of any weight loss program, a person will usually feel hunger pangs. Fennel can counter this feeling because it has a proven ability to reduce sugar cravings and suppress one's appetite. And as such, snacking on fennel seeds is a way to stay healthy and help a person in successfully making it through a diet program.

Chapter 10- Herbal Detox Herb- Marigold Flowers

If you are looking for an herb for a detox program, using marigold flowers is a wonderful option for you. With a reputation of being a natural skin healer, marigold has been proven to sooth indigestion and inflammation of the digestive tract. Also, it has the ability to support the detoxification process, thereby helping in the elimination of toxic matters that have accumulated in the human body over time.

By aiding cell renewal, the intestinal tract can be rebuilt with the use of marigold as an herbal detox herb. Apart from the digestive system, the gall bladder and the gut also benefit from this detoxifying agent. The flower heads of the bright yellow-orange marigolds is the source of the herbal components. The leaves and shoots are also being studied for active compounds that can be used for medicinal purposes.

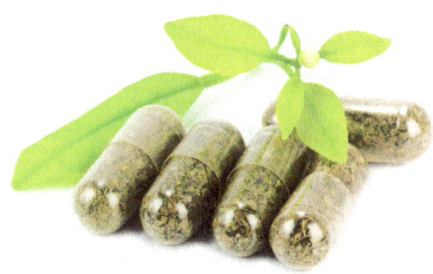

Where Can You Find Marigold?

Scientifically known as Calendula officinalis, marigold is grown in many parts of Canada and the United States. However, this annual plant is native to the eastern Mediterranean and southern Europe.

It is believed to originate in Egypt where it was highly valued for its rejuvenating properties. Marigold is also known as other names like pot marigold, garden marigold or calendula. These days, marigolds are often grown in home gardens in different countries all over the world.

How Can You Grow Marigold?

Marigolds are easy to grow as they can germinate freely in any kind of soil. The seeds are best sown in April because they prefer to grow under partial sun or sunny areas. The plants start to bear flowers in the month of June until winter frost kills them. Young plants will start to grow in spring if the seeds are allowed to scatter freely. They require no cultivation but when they grow too close, you have to thin out the plants in order for the branches to spread out. Also, you need to remove the weeds as they may disturb plant growth.

The most common uses of marigold herb include:

- Treatment for varicose veins
- Skin inflammation
- Leg ulcers
- Bedsores
- Promotes the healing of the skin
- Aids digestion and used as an antiseptic

It is important to note that marigolds may cause allergic reactions to some people. And when they are combined with other herbs, the effects may be altered resulting in unfavorable side effects. This herb is not advisable for pregnant women and breastfeeding mothers. So it is always best to consult your doctor before using any herbs for body detoxification.

David A. Grande

CHAPTER 11- HERBAL DETOX HERB-MILK THISTLE

Of the many methods used to detoxify the body, milk thistle is one of the herbs that have been given much attention. This natural herb is regarded as very effective in detoxifying the liver and in fact, it is one of the best there is. With the stressful activities of modern lifestyles and unhealthy foods or drinks that are bombarded with chemicals, it is very important that we take the necessary measures to improve our health, especially the condition of our liver.

Milk Thistle For Detoxifying The Liver

When used for detoxifying the body, milk thistle effectively strengthens the liver's external membranes. The protective layer that it forms around the liver serves as a protection that stops toxins from invading the cells, while at the same time promoting the regeneration of the cells that have been damaged. In addition, the antioxidant contents of milk thistle can help clean out free radicals caused by excessive alcohol intake.

These health benefits are not just simple claims from people who have used this herb. The herb's ability to cleanse the liver is documented extensively and medical studies have shown that it can offer beneficial effects on liver health. Some of the benefits when using milk thistle include:

- The reduction of the body's excessive hormone production
- Treatment of jaundice symptoms
- Liver rejuvenation

Apart from all the benefits mentioned, milk thistle is also good for people who are suffering from liver diseases like alcohol hepatitis, liver cirrhosis and hepatitis C.

How To Get Milk Thistle?

Milk thistle plant is not easy to grow. It is also not recommended for home use because extraction of the active chemical can only be done in alcohol. But those planning to use it for body detox need not worry, as much like the other herbs mentioned throughout this book; it is readily available in extract, tincture or capsule form.

How Does Milk Thistle Work?

In essence, the detox method that uses milk thistle starts at the intestine where the herb substances are being absorbed. The substances are then carried to the liver where they become concentrated. Therefore, the benefits of the herb's medicinal properties are best used by the liver cells. Most of these positive effects can be attributed to the silymarin compound which is highly concentrated in milk thistle.

However, the effectiveness of this herb may be lost when taken with certain medications like those used for seizures or general anesthesia. You may want to discuss taking milk thistle with a health provider first before using it for detox. This is especially true for those with allergic reactions to any plants belonging to the Daisy family.

David A. Grande

CHAPTER 12- HERBAL DETOX HERB-SPIRULINA

<u>What Is Spirulina?</u>

Spirulina is a blue-green algae that can be found in both fresh and sea water. It is primarily used as a dietary supplement for humans and can be bought in the market in the form of powder, flake and tablet. It is grown around the world and can be traced back in history as a food source for Mesoamericans like the Aztecs up to the 16th century. Today, it is produced commercially by Chile, Myanmar, Pakistan, China, India, Thailand, Taiwan and the United States.

<u>What Is Spirulina Used For?</u>

Due to the numerous beneficial enzymes contained in spirulina, it is proven to aid in many health conditions like anemia, visual problems, allergies and carbohydrate disorders. It is also a good aid in weight reduction because it is easier to digest than soy protein or meat despite the fact that it has 12 to 15 times more protein content. Apart from that, it is rich in beta carotene that can help support the natural defense of the body against sickness.

Spirulina is widely used in herbal detox because of its amazing properties.

1. The major benefit that it can offer is assisting and promoting the natural process of cleansing the body from the build-up of toxins.
2. It also helps in restoring diet deficiencies while boosting the body's metabolism at the same time. And when spirulina is taken after a rigorous exercise, the body will

recover faster and you will notice a remarkable improvement of your physical condition.

3. With Spirulina's ability to activate the natural defense mechanisms of the body, you will have an improved resistance against weakness, fatigue and disease. That's what makes spirulina ideal for a detox program because the body usually tends to feel weak and tired when it does not get the amount of food it usually consumes.

4. Spirulina is also highly recommended in detoxifying the body when you need to pass urine drug tests. It can effectively remove all chemicals and toxins from the urine, saliva, blood and hair of humans. With those qualities, it is a very helpful detox formula especially for those who are going to take medical exams as requirements for drivers' licenses, sports licenses, college admissions and as mandated by work places.

After taking spirulina for some time, the body will experience an alkalizing effect especially for the digestive system and the blood. It can help eliminate sugar cravings and other substances that humans can be addicted to. It can help achieve a balanced PH level in the body resulting in overall health and harmony in the functions of the vital organs.

CHAPTER 13- HERBAL DETOX HERB- WHITE SAGE

Scientifically known as Salvia apiana, white sage is an herb that grows naturally in the coastal areas of northwestern Mexico and the southwestern part of the United States. The stalks and leaves are the parts used for detoxification purposes.

Traditionally, white sage was used as a purifying agent for thousands of years. In the culture of Native Americans, the plant is believed to have a spiritual significance especially in calling the Great Spirit, purifying and uplifting the soul. Burnt white sage is claimed to cleanse the dormant energy from an object, a place or even a person. The smoke neutralizes the negative energies, thus leaving the body or the place reenergized and cleansed.

When used in rituals for cleansing, white sage can be made into a smudge stick by bundling the stalks together and tying at the bottom part. Another method used is by allowing the white sage to burn on charcoal then releasing the smoke that is used for purification.

The smoked loose leaf sprigs of white sage can also be used to prepare tea. When used as astringent for treating sore throats, the tea is best taken lukewarm. But if you want to use the tea as a stomach tonic, drinking it cold can do wonders.

The leaves are not only used for making tea. Rubbing crushed white sage leaves on the body can help eliminate body odor. The leaves are also used in making shampoo by some Native American tribes, not only for the purpose of cleaning the hair but also to prevent it from turning gray.

White sage can also be mixed with food, eaten raw or cooked. The ripened stem tops or the whole young stalks can be eaten raw. The seeds of white sage can also be toasted, ground into powder then mixed with cereals like oatmeal. The seeds can also be soaked in water all night and then taken as beverage or mixed with other fruit juices for added flavor.

In terms of medicinal properties, white sage is a plant that contains anti-spasmodic and expectorant properties. And due to these characteristics, the plant can be used to reduce mucus congestion and indigestion. And more importantly, the plant serves as a natural anti-septic that helps the human body in eliminating parasites and fungal infections. Other ailments that can benefit from the use of white sage include skin disorders, bad breath, excessive sweating, sore gums, and menstrual problems.

ABOUT THE AUTHOR

David A. Grande was always trying to find the right diet to help him to keep the weight off. When he discovered the 10 day detox diet he was skeptical at first but decided to give it a try. It started off slowly but soon he realized that it was a viable option to lose weight.

Based on the level of success that he had, he started to share with his family and close friends. The circle of persons that he was introducing this diet to grew and grew until he was fully entrenched in preparing informative pamphlets on the subject. That is how his book came into being.

CPSIA information can be obtained at www.ICGtesting.com
Printed in the USA
LVOW01s2256050815

449051LV00016B/385/P